ALOE VERA FOR BEGINNERS

Unlocking Aloe Vera's Healing Power A
Comprehensive Guide To Nature's Miracle Plant,
Health, Beauty, And Wellness

Georgette Lockett

DISCLAIMER

The author of this book is not affiliated, associated, endorsed, sponsored, or approved by any company or individual. The views and opinions expressed in this book are solely those of the author and do not necessarily reflect the official policy or position of any entity.

The author hereby disclaims any relationship, collaboration, or partnership with any company or individual mentioned in this book. Any references to products, services, or individuals are provided for informational purposes only and should not be construed as an endorsement or recommendation.

Readers are advised to exercise their own judgment and discretion when applying the information provided in this book. The author shall not be held responsible for any actions taken by readers based on the content of this book.

This book is intended for general informational purposes only, and the author makes no representations or warranties of any kind, express or implied, about the completeness, accuracy, reliability, suitability, or availability of the information contained herein. Any reliance on the information in this book is at the reader's own risk.

The author reserves the right to update, change, or modify any information in this book without notice. It is the responsibility of the reader to verify any information before taking any actions based on the content of this book.

By reading this book, the reader acknowledges and agrees to the terms of this disclaimer.

Table of Contents

INTRODUCTION

Overview of Aloe Vera

Aloe Vera, technically known as Aloe barbadensis miller, is a succulent plant that belongs to the genus Aloe. Renowned for its therapeutic and cosmetic benefits, Aloe Vera has a long history of human usage, stretching back thousands of years. The plant is native to the Arabian Peninsula but is currently grown in numerous places worldwide, due to its varied usage.

Historical Significance

The historical relevance of Aloe Vera may be traced back to ancient civilizations. The plant's medicinal benefits were well-recognized in ancient Egyptian, Greek, Roman, and Indian societies. Egyptians referred to it as the "plant of immortality," stressing its claimed healing qualities.

Throughout history, Aloe Vera has been a mainstay in traditional medicine, making its way into cures for skin illnesses, stomach difficulties, and more.

Importance In Traditional And Modern Uses

Aloe Vera's value transcends both traditional and contemporary usage. In traditional medicine, it has been employed for healing wounds, skin irritations, and stomach disorders. Its gel, derived from the inside leaf, is a traditional cure for burns and skin disorders. In current times, Aloe Vera is an important element in several sectors, including medicines, cosmetics, and food. Its broad usage in skincare products, drinks, and supplements highlights its enduring importance in modern health and wellbeing.

CHAPTER 1

Botanical Background

Taxonomy And Classification

Aloe Vera, technically known as Aloe barbadensis miller, belongs to the Asphodelaceae family and is a perennial, succulent plant noted for its therapeutic and medicinal characteristics. Taxonomically, it comes within the order Asparagales and the genus Aloe. The Aloe genus comprises a varied variety of plants, but Aloe Vera stands out for its extensive usage in numerous civilizations spanning ages.

Morphology And Structure

Aloe Vera is defined by its distinctive shape and succulent nature. The plant often exhibits thick, meaty, lance-shaped leaves that grow in rosette patterns. The leaves contain a gel-like material that is commonly exploited for its therapeutic benefits.

The outside surface of the leaves has a green color, while the inside gel is clear and mucilaginous.

Its root structure is rather shallow, responding well to dry circumstances. This succulent perennial demonstrates CAM (Crassulacean Acid Metabolism) photosynthesis, enabling it to effectively save water in dry settings.

Habitat And Cultivation

Aloe Vera is native to the Arabian Peninsula but is currently farmed in numerous subtropical and tropical places worldwide, considering its resilience to varying conditions. It thrives in well-drained, sandy soil and needs minimum water, making it appropriate for desert regions. However, it may also thrive in pots inside under ideal circumstances.

Cultivation procedures for Aloe Vera entail supplying enough sunshine, particularly in semi-arid to arid areas. Excessive wetness may lead to root rot, underlining the importance of well-draining soil. Propagation generally happens by offsets or pups generated by older plants, easing its cultivation procedure.

The commercial production of Aloe Vera entails specialized measures to maintain maximum growth and quality, typically focused on organic approaches to preserve the potency of its medicinal ingredients.

Understanding the botanical origins of Aloe Vera lays the context for grasping its many uses and importance in traditional, alternative, and contemporary applications.

CHAPTER 2

Nutritional Composition

Aloe Vera, a succulent plant belonging to the Aloe genus, features a diverse variety of ingredients that contribute to its medicinal and nutritional benefits.

Chemical Constituents

• **Polysaccharides:** A significant constituent, polysaccharides such as acemannan, glucomannans, and polymannans, are key components contributing to the plant's therapeutic benefits. Acemannan, especially, has exhibited immunostimulatory properties.

• **Anthraquinones:** Aloin and emodin are among the bioactive anthraquinones contained in Aloe Vera. They exhibit laxative characteristics but are often eliminated or decreased in commercially made products because of their possible harmful effects.

- **Sterols:** Beta-sitosterol, campesterol, and lupeol are sterols contained in Aloe Vera, contributing to its anti-inflammatory and cholesterol-lowering qualities.

- **Enzymes:** Aloe Vera includes numerous enzymes such as amylase, bradykinase, lipase, and catalase, which promote digestion and offer anti-inflammatory qualities.

- **Vitamins:** It includes vitamins like A, C, E, B1, B2, B3, B6, and B12, aiding to skin health, immunity, and general well-being.

- **Minerals:** Aloe Vera includes vital minerals such as calcium, magnesium, zinc, chromium, selenium, and potassium, which play critical roles in numerous physiological activities.

Vitamins, Minerals, And Enzymes

- **Vitamins:** Aloe Vera's vitamin content adds greatly to its health advantages. Vitamin A improves skin health, eyesight, and immunological function, while vitamins C and E work as antioxidants, boosting the immune system and skin health. B vitamins are required for energy generation as well as general metabolic function.

- **Minerals:** The presence of minerals, especially calcium and magnesium, aids in bone health and the operation of the muscular and neurological systems. Potassium is necessary for fluid balance and heart health, while zinc is required for immune function and wound healing.

- **Enzymes:** The enzymes included in Aloe Vera aid in a variety of metabolic processes. Amylase helps with carbohydrate digestion, lipase helps with fat digestion, and bradykinase adds to its anti-inflammatory qualities by lowering swelling.

Health Benefits Of Aloe Vera Components

• **Skin Health:** Aloe Vera's contents, such as vitamins C and E, as well as polysaccharides, provide moisturizing, soothing, and healing capabilities, assisting in the treatment of burns, wounds, and numerous skin disorders such as psoriasis and acne.

• **Digestive Health:** Enzymes such as amylase and lipase aid digestion, possibly alleviating gastrointestinal problems. The calming characteristics of aloe vera may help relieve symptoms of acid reflux or irritable bowel syndrome.

• **Immune Support:** Aloe Vera's polysaccharides and antioxidants may help the immune system by increasing cellular activity and eliminating free radicals.

Understanding Aloe Vera's nutritional makeup provides insight into its many therapeutic uses and prepares the way for its beneficial features to be used in a variety of disciplines, including medicine, cosmetics, and dietary supplements.

CHAPTER 3

Medicinal Properties

Healing And Therapeutic Uses

The healing powers and therapeutic uses of Aloe Vera, a succulent plant species with a long history of medical usage, are renowned.

Aloe Vera's therapeutic potential covers a wide range of disciplines, due principally to its vast array of bioactive chemicals. It is well known for its skin-related therapeutic properties. The transparent, gel-like fluid derived from its leaves includes polysaccharides, including acemannan, which have immunomodulatory characteristics and promote wound healing and tissue repair. This gel is often used topically to treat small burns, wounds, abrasions, and sunburns, offering soothing comfort and promoting speedier healing.

Its antibacterial capabilities also aid in the prevention of wound infections.

Anti-Inflammatory And Antioxidant Effects

The anti-inflammatory and antioxidant properties of aloe vera are mostly ascribed to substances such as bradykinase, salicylic acid, and other enzymes. These components reduce inflammation and relieve pain linked with illnesses such as arthritis and dermatitis. Furthermore, its high antioxidant content, which includes vitamins C and E, flavonoids, and polyphenols, aids in the neutralization of free radicals, lowering oxidative stress and strengthening the body's defense against chronic illnesses and aging.

Skin And Wound Care Applications

Aloe Vera's effectiveness in skincare goes beyond wound healing. It is a common component in cosmetics, lotions, and creams because of its moisturizing and calming effects. It effectively penetrates the skin, moisturizing and nourishing it while assisting in the treatment of numerous dermatological conditions such as acne, psoriasis, and eczema. The natural cooling impact of the gel relieves skin irritation and itching.

This chapter highlights the plant's diverse therapeutic potential, demonstrating its efficacy in treating a variety of skin diseases and emphasizing its anti-inflammatory and antioxidant characteristics, which contribute to general health and well-being.

CHAPTER 4

Aloe Vera In Traditional Medicine

Historical Uses Across Cultures

Aloe Vera has a long history that is strongly ingrained in traditional medicine from numerous countries. Its medical powers and therapeutic uses have been known for millennia.

The plant's medicinal virtues have been recorded in ancient Egyptian, Greek, Roman, Chinese, Indian, and Arabian civilizations. It was regarded as the "plant of immortality" in Egypt and was often represented in murals in pharaoh tombs, emphasizing its value. Its usage for wound healing and digestive disorders was recognized by Greek and Roman doctors such as Dioscorides and Pliny the Elder. Aloe Vera was recognized by Traditional Chinese Medicine (TCM) for its cooling effects and use for skin diseases.

Aloe Vera was valued for its various therapeutic qualities throughout these different civilizations.

Folk Remedies And Cultural Practices

Aloe Vera has been utilized in folk remedies for healing skin diseases, burns, wounds, and digestive issues around the globe. It was also used for internal cleaning and as a digestive aid in certain cultures. Aloe Vera was included in traditional healing procedures by indigenous people, who attributed it to spiritual and medical importance.

Global Influence On Traditional Healing

Aloe Vera's reputation as a healing plant has crossed geographical borders, resulting in its incorporation into traditional healing techniques all around the globe. The plant's reach and reputation extended as trade routes developed, solidifying its role in traditional medicine across continents.

Understanding the history of Aloe Vera's use in many cultures gives insights into its enormous effect on traditional medicinal techniques. Its voyage through time demonstrates not only its medical adaptability but also its cultural value and the confidence that many communities have in its healing abilities.

CHAPTER 5

Modern Applications

Commercial Uses In Cosmetics And Skincare

Because of its strong moisturizing characteristics and skin-friendly components, Aloe Vera is widely used in cosmetics. Its gel is used in a variety of skincare products, such as lotions, creams, and sunscreens.

The plant's ability to treat skin irritations and moderate burns, paired with its moisturizing quality, makes it a suitable component in beauty and cosmetic formulas. The inclusion of Aloe Vera in shampoos and conditioners also offers nutrients to the hair and scalp, assisting in the maintenance of healthy hair.

Aloe Vera In Pharmaceuticals

Aloe Vera's therapeutic benefits extend to pharmaceutical uses. Its anti-inflammatory, antibacterial, and wound-healing properties make it an important ingredient in a variety of pharmacological treatments. It is used to make ointments, gels, and creams to treat small wounds, burns, and skin irritations. Furthermore, because of its ability to enhance digestive health, it has been used in several laxatives and digestive supplements.

Role In Nutraceuticals And Health Products

Aloe Vera has made its way into nutraceuticals and health goods. Because of its extensive nutritional profile, which includes vitamins, enzymes, and antioxidants, Aloe Vera-based supplements and beverages have been developed. These products often promise to help with digestion, immunological support, and general well-being.

The use of the gel in the form of beverages or capsules is thought to provide a variety of health benefits.

Aloe Vera is widely used in contemporary applications owing to its many advantages and adaptability. Its usage in a wide range of sectors, from cosmetics to medicines and nutraceuticals, demonstrates its enormous potential and ongoing research into novel applications and formulations. The possibility for new uses of Aloe Vera in numerous areas is projected to rise as research advances, further strengthening its place in contemporary businesses.

CHAPTER 6

Aloe Vera Cultivation And Processing

Cultivation Techniques And Conditions

Aloe Vera flourishes in dry and semi-arid settings because of its hardiness. This succulent requires particular cultivation procedures. Outdoors, the plant may be cultivated in areas with well-drained sandy or loamy soil and a warm, dry environment. It is also grown inside, allowing for more regulated settings. Temperature, humidity, and enough sunshine are examples of controlled circumstances.

Aloe Vera takes little water and is tolerant to a wide range of soil types, although it requires adequate drainage to avoid root rot. Commercially, it is often cultivated on raised beds or containers to properly regulate moisture levels.

Harvesting And Processing Methods

Harvesting Aloe Vera entails carefully extracting the gel from its leaves. Harvesting mature leaves, generally older than three years, is done. The exterior green rind is peeled away, revealing the interior gel. The gel may be retrieved either manually or mechanically, assuring cleanliness and reducing contamination.

Filtration, stabilization, and preservation of the gel are all phases of the processing process. Filtration is used to eliminate any particles or residues. Stabilization seeks to preserve the integrity of bioactive substances by reducing oxidation and enzymatic breakdown. Refrigeration or the use of natural preservatives, for example, aids in the preservation of the gel's freshness and efficacy.

Quality Control And Standardization

To assure the potency and safety of the finished product, quality control in Aloe Vera manufacturing is critical. Monitoring cultivation procedures, assuring the absence of pesticides or pollutants, and analyzing the purity and concentration of beneficial substances are all part of this process.

The goal of standardization methods is to set and maintain particular quality characteristics, such as polysaccharide, acemannan, vitamin, and mineral content. This provides uniformity between batches and goods, allowing customers to get the advantages intended.

Standards and criteria for Aloe Vera products are often enforced by regulatory organizations, contributing to customer safety and product dependability.

Aloe Vera is processed in a variety of ways for diverse uses such as gels, juices, powders, and extracts. Each technique is designed to maintain its positive characteristics while delivering the necessary effectiveness.

Producers may manufacture high-quality Aloe Vera products with better effectiveness and safety by understanding and improving cultivation and processing procedures, satisfying the needs of diverse sectors such as cosmetics, medicines, and nutraceuticals.

CHAPTER 7

Aloe Vera Products

Because of its adaptable nature and significant medicinal capabilities, aloe vera finds its way into a wide variety of goods. This chapter goes into the wide spectrum of aloe vera formulations and products.

Extracts, Gels, Juices, And Concentrates

Aloe Vera Gel: Aloe vera gel, produced from the inner leaf, is one of the most popular and frequently used products. The soothing, hydrating, and cooling characteristics of the gel make it a skincare mainstay. Topically, it is used to treat burns, wounds, sunburns, and skin irritations.

Aloe Vera Juice: Made from the aloe leaf, this juice includes a variety of bioactive substances such as polysaccharides, antioxidants, and enzymes.

When used orally, it is said to provide internal advantages such as easing digestion, improving immunity, and supporting general well-being.

Concentrates and Extracts: Aloe vera extract or juice concentrates are utilized in a variety of formulations, including creams, lotions, ointments, and nutritional supplements. These concentrated versions maintain the bioactive components, allowing for a wide range of surface and interior uses.

Supplements And Formulations

Aloe vera is a frequent element in nutritional supplements such as capsules and powders. These supplements often seek to improve digestive health, boost the immune system, or provide antioxidant effects. They might include concentrated aloe extracts or gel.

Topical Formulations: Aloe vera is widely used in the skincare and cosmetic sectors in formulations such as moisturizers, cleansers, shampoos, and conditioners. Its inherent moisturizing characteristics make it an appealing substance for skin and hair care.

Market Trends And Consumer Preferences

Consumer Demand is Growing: The worldwide market for aloe vera products has grown significantly as a result of growing consumer knowledge of natural cures and a demand for sustainable, plant-based solutions in personal care and wellbeing.

Quality and Authenticity: As consumers become more sophisticated, they seek high-quality, pure aloe vera products. Purchase choices are heavily influenced by authenticity, purity, and certificates validating organic agriculture and processing practices.

Trends and Innovations: New product creation is fueled by ongoing research and invention. Eco-friendly packaging, formulas with fewer synthetic ingredients, and a focus on cruelty-free, sustainable practices are all on the rise.

Customization and adaptation: Aloe vera products appeal to a wide range of demographics, resulting in tailored formulas for particular applications or consumer groups. Individual preferences, such as natural, organic, or allergic items, are met by this personalization.

The diverse range of aloe vera products illustrates the plant's adaptability and broad adoption in a variety of businesses. As consumer tastes shift toward natural and sustainable solutions, the demand for high-quality aloe vera products is expected to remain strong, spurring greater innovation in formulations and uses. Understanding customer preferences and maintaining quality standards will continue to be critical for the worldwide success and expansion of aloe vera-based goods.

CHAPTER 8

Clinical Studies And Research

Scientific Investigations

Aloe vera has been the subject of various scientific studies looking at its possible health benefits. Its chemical ingredients, modes of action and diverse uses have all been studied by researchers. This research varies from laboratory tests to clinical trials, to reveal the whole range of its therapeutic qualities.

Clinical Trials And Findings

Aloe vera clinical trials have focused on a variety of health issues, including skin ailments, gastrointestinal disorders, wound healing, and more. Aloe vera gel has been studied for its usefulness in treating burns, dermatitis, psoriasis, and other skin problems.

Furthermore, studies on the benefits of aloe vera on digestive disorders such as irritable bowel syndrome (IBS) and ulcerative colitis have been done.

Emerging Discoveries And Areas Of Study

Aloe vera research is always revealing new aspects of its potential. Emerging research is looking at its immunomodulatory activities, possible anticancer capabilities, and influence on metabolic diseases such as diabetes and obesity. Scientists are also investigating its function in dental care and its impact on oral health, to reduce periodontal disorders.

Furthermore, as technology progresses, investigations on innovative formulations and delivery technologies to improve the bioavailability and performance of aloe vera-based products are being conducted. The synergy between aloe vera and other natural substances is also a growing field of study, with researchers looking at possible enhanced advantages when paired with other herbal medicines or pharmaceutical drugs.

In conclusion, research into the different qualities of aloe vera has shown encouraging findings in a variety of sectors. Aloe vera is a versatile plant with enormous promise for human health and well-being, from its historical usage in traditional medicine to its modern applications in cosmetics, medicines, and nutraceuticals.

The plant's methods of action, therapeutic potential, and safety profiles have all been improved because of extensive scientific research. Clinical investigations have supported various traditional applications of aloe vera while also revealing new areas where it might be useful. As continuous research uncovers its qualities, the future offers bright opportunities for innovative formulations, wider medicinal uses, and a deeper understanding of how to maximize its health advantages.

The extensive nutritional profile of aloe vera, together with its many bioactive components, makes a strong argument for its further investigation in medicine and related disciplines. Nonetheless, despite its promising characteristics, judicious cultivation, processing, standardization, and quality control remain critical to realize its full potential and assure customer safety and effectiveness in diverse products.

In summary, aloe vera's path from ancient therapeutic traditions to current scientific examination demonstrates its lasting importance in supporting health and wellbeing. Aloe vera's adaptability, supported by scientific data, establishes it as a significant botanical resource set to play an increasingly vital role in varied industries, helping mankind in a variety of ways.

CHAPTER 9

Aloe Vera In Holistic Health

Integrative Medicine Approaches

Aloe Vera has found a large role in integrative medicine, a science that integrates traditional medical treatments with alternative medicines. Its adaptable qualities, including anti-inflammatory, wound-healing, and antioxidant capabilities, have made it a beneficial component in a variety of integrative medicine techniques. Aloe Vera is often used by integrative practitioners to supplement traditional therapy.

Holistic Health And Aloe Vera

Aloe Vera has a varied function in holistic health. Its advantages go beyond physical health and include mental, emotional, and spiritual well-being. Holistic practitioners stress the interdependence of all areas of health and see Aloe Vera as a holistic medicine that may help with overall well-being. Its use is consistent with the holistic approach to health, which strives to balance the body, mind, and spirit for maximum health.

Lifestyle Applications And Practices

Aloe Vera has been used in a variety of lifestyle activities that promote health and well-being. It is present in many parts of everyday living, from nutritional supplements to skincare procedures. Some people use Aloe Vera pills in their diets because of the stated digestive advantages and possibly immune-boosting characteristics. Furthermore, because of its moisturizing, soothing, and renewing benefits on the skin, it is often used in skincare and cosmetic routines.

Aloe Vera is often utilized in holistic practices with other natural medicines such as herbal supplements, meditation, yoga, and mindfulness methods to promote a holistic approach to health. Its presence in these activities reflects the concept that a balanced lifestyle that includes physical, mental, and emotional components is necessary for general well-being.

Aloe Vera is popular among holistic health advocates not just for its physical health advantages, but also for its possible contributions to mental clarity, emotional balance, and spiritual alignment. Its natural characteristics are said to work in tandem with the body's inherent healing processes, harmonizing with the holistic perspective that sees health as a state of balance and harmony across numerous dimensions.

Aloe Vera's adaptability and prospective benefits to holistic health are still being investigated by practitioners and academics attempting to improve overall well-being via a complete and integrated approach that includes the mind, body, and spirit.

CHAPTER 10

Sustainability And Future Prospects

Environmental Impact

Because of the popularity of aloe vera, commercial cultivation has increased, drawing attention to its environmental effect. Farming and processing on a large scale may put a burden on natural resources, altering soil quality, water consumption, and biodiversity. To reduce these consequences, sustainable behaviors are critical. Eco-friendly practices such as organic farming, integrated pest control, and water-efficient irrigation assist to reduce the environmental impact.

Sustainable Farming Practices

Adopting approaches that maintain ecosystems, promote biodiversity, and reduce resource depletion is required for Aloe Vera agriculture to be sustainable. Cropping rotation, intercropping with suitable species, and the use of natural fertilizers increase soil fertility while decreasing dependence on chemical inputs. Water usage is reduced by practices such as rainwater collecting and efficient irrigation systems.

In addition, sustainable harvesting procedures promote plant regeneration and ecological equilibrium. Aloe Vera populations are protected from overexploitation by strategies such as selective harvesting and regulated extraction processes.

Future Trends And Innovations

1. **Research and Development:** Ongoing scientific research is uncovering novel medicinal characteristics and uses for Aloe Vera. Future advancements in medicine, cosmetics, and nutraceuticals will be driven by research into new chemicals and their potential benefits.

2. Biotechnological Advances: Biotechnology provides prospective options for increasing Aloe Vera production, increasing active component concentrations, and improving product quality. Genetic research might contribute to the development of disease-resistant cultivars or the optimization of growth under a variety of environmental circumstances.

3. Market Expansion: The growing demand for natural and organic goods drives the Aloe Vera market. Formulation, packaging, and delivery system innovations respond to changing customer demands, broadening its reach across sectors.

4. Sustainability Initiatives: Stricter legislation and customer awareness push companies to adopt more environmentally friendly methods. Fairtrade, ethical sourcing and eco-certification initiatives support responsible Aloe Vera farming and processing.

5. Collaboration: Collaborations between academic institutions, industrial actors, and local communities may promote long-term progress. Collaborative programs concentrating on conservation, eco-friendly techniques, and community welfare help to make the Aloe Vera sector more sustainable.

Aloe Vera's future depends on combining economic interests with environmental management. Implementing sustainable techniques not only assures the long-term viability of Aloe Vera agriculture but also helps to preserve ecosystems and assist local populations. Continuous research and new tactics will ensure its relevance across a wide range of industries while protecting the planet's resources for future generations.

Conclusion

Aloe Vera is a unique plant that has captivated human attention for ages because of its rich history, various uses, and multiple health benefits. This conclusion tries to highlight the important elements mentioned during the Aloe Vera inquiry, offering insights into its relevance as well as prospective areas for future research.

Summary Of Aloe Vera's Significance

Throughout the investigation of Aloe Vera, it becomes clear that this succulent plant is very important in a variety of disciplines. It has long been recognized for its medicinal powers, with uses in traditional medicine throughout countries. Aloe Vera has long been used to promote health and well-being, from wound healing to skin care.

The botanical history of Aloe Vera, which was reviewed in Chapter 1, focused on its taxonomy, morphology, and habitat, offering a core knowledge of the plant. The second chapter delves into the nutritional content, clarifying the myriad of chemical elements, vitamins, minerals, and enzymes that contribute to its health advantages.

The medicinal characteristics were fully investigated in Chapter 3, highlighting its anti-inflammatory and antioxidant actions, making it a mainstay in a variety of therapeutic applications.

As stated in Chapter 5, recent uses of Aloe Vera indicate its broad usage in cosmetics, medicines, and nutraceuticals. The production and processing of Aloe Vera, as described in Chapter 6, highlight the need to use sustainable techniques to ensure the quality of Aloe Vera products. Chapter 7 gave information on the many Aloe Vera products on the market, ranging from extracts and gels to juices and concentrates.

Scientific research and clinical trials, as described in Chapter 8, have greatly added to our knowledge of Aloe Vera's effectiveness. The results confirm its conventional usage while also opening up new areas for investigation, pointing to possible benefits in a variety of health issues.

Potential Areas For Further Research

While there is a considerable corpus of study on Aloe Vera, there are still areas that deserve additional investigation. Future research should focus on the processes behind its healing capabilities, the unique interactions between its components and biological systems, and its potential in innovative therapeutic approaches. Furthermore, thorough scientific studies might give useful insights into the influence of Aloe Vera on certain health issues.

Finally, Aloe Vera is a botanical miracle with a rich history and a bright future. Its adaptability to a wide range of uses, from ancient medicine to contemporary cosmetics and medicines, demonstrates its adaptability. Aloe Vera remains a source of intrigue and possible breakthroughs as we traverse the difficulties of sustainable agricultural techniques, market trends, and developing technologies.

The voyage through the chapters has shown Aloe Vera's complex character, underlining its significance not just as a botanical wonder but also as a source of practical advantages for human health and well-being. The continuing investigation of Aloe Vera's potential offers the prospect of unlocking new dimensions in medicine, agriculture, and environmental sustainability as we move ahead. Aloe Vera unquestionably has a significant and lasting position in the tapestry of botanical miracles.

THE END

60